THE LOW-SODIUM RECIPES COOKBOOK FOR SENIORS

Healthy and Nourishing Low-Salt Dishes to Manage Heart Disease and Blood Pressure

TABLE OF CONTENT

TABLE OF CONTENT

INTRODUCTION

Sodium is an essential part of everyone's diet, the human body could not function without it. However, there can be too much of a good thing. Americans tend to overdo it on sodium, which can contribute to many health issues, including high blood pressure and heart disease. However, it is not always easy to know what sodium is in and how much you are consuming.

Sodium is a mineral that your body must have in order to function properly. The primary source of dietary sodium is sodium chloride, or salt, more than three-quarters of which comes from processed foods. Although sodium is vital to a number of routine body functions, too much can have adverse effects, particularly for people who are sensitive to sodium. Excessive sodium can cause hypertension, which in turn can lead to other health problems.

Sodium is a mineral that carries an electrical charge, known as an electrolyte. Electrolytes facilitate muscle contraction and nerve cell transmission.

Ions of sodium, potassium and chloride trigger muscle contractions and nerve impulses when they shift places across cell membranes. A nerve cell at rest has positively charged potassium ions inside the cell and is surrounded outside the cell by positively charged sodium ions and negatively charged chloride ions. When stimulated, potassium ions rush out of the cell as sodium ions rush in, creating an electrical signal or nerve impulse. A similar scenario occurs during the contraction of muscles.

CHAPTER ONE

COOKING HACK TO USE SALT

Salt enhances the natural flavors in food, so it's no wonder we love it so much! And it's found in about everything from potato chips and pretzels, to raw chicken and turkey, to chocolate chip cookies. This makes it incredibly hard to reduce for those of us who need to! Cooking at home is the best way to control the amount of salt you eat, because the majority of the salt we consume doesn't come from the salt shaker! It's already in the food we eat.

The recommendation for sodium intake for healthy people is less than 2300 mg per day. Ideally, we should all be consuming less than 1500 mg sodium per day.

If you have high blood pressure, you should definitely be working to keep your sodium intake below that. But don't we need sodium? Yes. Sodium is an electrolyte (like potassium), and it is necessary to help keep the body functioning normally.

The human body requires about 500 mg of sodium for normal functioning daily. Some people need more; those who exercise or sweat a lot, like I said an average American consumes in excess of 3400 mg daily, so most people are in no danger of not getting enough for the body to work right. Most all foods naturally contain some sodium, so even if you never added any salt at all, you'd probably be fine.

The best way to determine how much sodium you eat is by keeping track of it. People are notoriously inaccurate with estimates of how much they eat, and not all foods with a lot of sodium taste salty. It's important to take a look at labels on all the foods and beverages you consume. Writing it down is most helpful.

How can you Cook with Less Salt? Salt makes your food taste good, but consuming too much of it can sometimes cause high blood pressure which can ultimately lead to other health issues.

I know you are facing this reality and I have a message for you: You're not doomed to tasteless food. The beauty of home cooking is that you're in control, and there are lots of creative ways to add flavor, while also avoiding excess salt. I will show you the tricks and techniques that'll reset your cooking habits.

Know Your Salt

Table Salt

This tiny, refined salt has uniform granules and is often used for everyday cooking, baking and as a table condiment. A teaspoon of table salt will be saltier than a teaspoon of coarse kosher salt. This is because the granules of table salt are smaller and denser, so you wind up with more of them in a teaspoon. Morton's is probably the most recognizable brand of table salt. It may or may not have iodine added. Iodine is a mineral that helps prevent hypothyroidism, but some dislike the faintly metallic taste it adds. And luckily, our diets in the United States are rich enough in natural iodine that we don't need it added to our salt anymore, so you can buy the type without.

Coarse Kosher Salt

With bigger granules that vary in size and texture, coarse kosher salt is often used for seasoning meat, brining solutions, topping pretzels and breads, rimming cocktail glasses and salting pasta water. It's great for cooking because it dissolves quickly, and it has lower salinity than table salt. Kosher salt is used for koshering meat in accordance with Jewish dietary laws, so it's additive free and has a clean taste. Diamond Crystal and Morton's kosher are the brands you're most likely to find at your local grocery. Keep in mind that even the same kind of salt can vary by brand. For example, Morton's kosher salt is actually saltier than Diamond due to the production method.

Sea Salt

From flaky to coarse, this type of salt varies in granule size, texture and color, depending on where it's from and how it's processed. Flaky sea salt is typically used as a flavor finisher due to its delicate, crunchy texture (and high price). Maldon is perhaps the most widely available brand of flaky sea salt or look for salts labeled "fleur de sel" or "sel gris." (Note, sel gris is processed a little differently from Maldon and fleur de sel but can be used in the same way, i.e. as a finisher.) Try adding it on salads or as a finishing flourish on indulgent chocolate and caramel desserts for a perfect balance of salty and sweet. Refined sea salt can be used the way you'd use coarse kosher salt in everyday cooking and baking. It's granules range in size from medium to fine. This type of sea salt is also relatively inexpensive because it's easier to produce (sea water is boiled down) than labor-intensive flaky sea salt (harvested from saltwater beds near the ocean).

Counter-intuitively, you might find yourself buying more salt or rather, a different kind of salt when you embark on lower-sodium diet. If you don't already keep either kosher or a refined sea salt on hand, I would highly recommend picking up one of these less-salty salts for cooking and baking. And salt is not the only way to flavor your food, which brings us to the next point.

Add Flavor (Not Salt!)

When you set down the saltshaker, you set yourself on a path to more creative cooking. The ingredients and techniques described below will help you add new flavor dimensions to your cooking.

- Acid: Add some tangy contrast to your dish with a splash lemon or lime juice or a dash of your favorite flavored vinegar, like apple cider, white wine or balsamic.

- Aromatics: Garlic, ginger, onions, shallots and even lemon or lime zest, all of these ingredients add flavor that will bring your dish to life.

- Browning: Your meat turns out deeply flavorful when you cook it over high heat until a crust forms on the outside.

- Caramelization: Sautéing mushrooms or onions until they turn dark brown adds incredible richness and sweetness to anything you're cooking.

- Fresh herbs: Give your dish a bright garnish with a sprinkle of soft herbs, like parsley, basil, mint or cilantro. Or, add sturdier herbs, like rosemary and oregano, before cooking for an additional layer of flavor.

- Heat: From fruity calabrians to smoky chipotles and fiery chiles de arbol, a little bit of chili is an easy way to amp up the flavor of your dish.

- Sauces or condiments: When in doubt, a sauce it could be anything from salad dressing, mayo, gremolata, barbecue sauce or even ketchup, is a surefire way to take your dish to the next level. If you start from scratch, you'll know exactly how much salt you're adding.

Keep these tips in mind; knowing how to add a splash of flavor will help you find ways to modify secretly salty foods, so you can keep enjoying them.

Beware of Secretly Salty Foods

Have heard a lot about added sugar these days but added salt is also something to be aware of. The more you know about where salt is being added to your foods, the better you'll get at avoiding it.

Meats, poultry and seafood: It's the added salt that you might not be aware of here. Saltwater or saline solutions are used to enhance flavor or to help with preservation. Be sure to check the package information, look at the sodium amounts and how much of your recommended daily intake they represent, before purchasing.

Additionally, some meats are pre-seasoned or pre-sauced, it's best to skip these and season yourself if you're cutting back on sodium. Finally, don't forget about cold cuts and cured meats, which tend to be high in sodium. Again, reading labels is important.

Cheese: You're probably aware that salt is a key component of cheese, but did you know that it's especially key in hard cheeses, like Parmesan and soft-rind cheeses, like Brie? When you're looking for a snacking or cooking cheese, search out lower-sodium options like mozzarella, ricotta or goat cheese.

Store-bought baked goods: Salt makes sweets sweeter, which is why it's often called for in recipes for cookies and other baked goods. In addition, butter can be sweet or salted. Bake your own treats and you won't have to worry about added salt in your cookies or cakes.

Savory snacks and nuts: Trail mix and nuts can be a wholesome snacking option, especially when you make your own mix or buy nuts that aren't seasoned (salt and salty ingredients often play a large role in seasoning nuts). Toasting nuts can add flavor, as can mixing in various types of spices. Relying on these methods of increasing flavor and you can reduce the amount of salt used.

Spice rubs: Making your own is an easy way to control the amount of salt used. It's also a fun way to get creative in the kitchen, and you might be surprised at all you can make with what's already in your spice cabinet. Get started with these six essential spice rubs.

You don't necessarily have to cut out the foods above, but you might want to consider enjoying them at home where you're in charge of ingredients and able to prepare them in a way that suits your diet.

TRICKS FOR REDUCING SALT

Know that your taste buds will adjust to your new lower salt way of cooking. It will take about 7-10 days. Keep trying new things! Don't salt your food as you cook. If a recipe calls for salt, omit it. Taste your food after you put it on your plate, and add a little salt then if you think it needs it.

Rinse your canned goods. Beans, vegetables and tuna are preserved in liquids that are often very salty. A quick rinse before combining with other ingredients will help remove some of the added salt.

Season and taste as you cook. This is a foolproof way to see the impact of various ingredients and get your taste buds accustomed to different salt levels. (Remember, kosher and sea salt are great to use in cooking as they dissolve quickly and are less salty than table salt.)

Premeasure super-salty condiments, like soy sauce, rather than blindly sprinkling on your food. Better yet, integrate these types of condiments into the dish or sauce. Not only will this help you keep a handle on how much you're using, you might also discover that a little goes a long way.

Buy lower or reduced-sodium versions of your pantry staples. Broth, salad dressing, canned soup, condiments and other packaged goods are commonly available in lower or reduced-sodium forms these days.

Find a no-salt seasoning blend that you like. There's more than one option on the market and these blends can really save a meal.

Start with half the seasoning packet when making a shortcut meal from a box or mixing up a salad dressing from a packet. You can always add more, if the taste is falling flat. But you might discover that you really don't need the whole packet. So now that you know how to season your food to suit your tastes and meet your dietary needs, it's time to get cooking! Get started with a couple of our best lower-sodium recipes below.

CHAPTER TWO

LOW-SODIUM RECIPES

Raspberry Spinach Salad with Caramelized Masala Pumpkin Seeds
TOTAL TIME: 25 MINUTES

INGREDIENTS

- 8 ounces of washed baby spinach, 8 cups
- 8 ounces raspberries, 3 cups, washed and drained
- 1 large ripe avocado, peeled, pitted, and cubed
- 2 Tablespoons white balsamic vinegar
- 4 Tablespoons extra virgin olive oil
- sea salt to taste
- optional touch of maple syrup if your vinegar is really sour
- 1/2 cup raw pumpkin seeds
- 1 Teaspoon garam masala
- 1 Tablespoon maple syrup
- sea salt to taste, I used 1/4 Teaspoon

DIRECTIONS

- Place the baby spinach, raspberries, and avocado in a large serving bowl.

- Place the ingredients for the white balsamic into a glass jar, secure the lid, and shake the dressing together until it's emulsified. Season to taste with sea salt and a touch of maple syrup if needed. If the dressing separates before you're ready to use it, simply shake it together again.

- Toast the pumpkin seeds in a 9" cast iron pan over medium-low heat for 10 minutes, or until the pumpkins seeds smell fragrantly toasted, and they start to make small popping sounds.

- Add the garam masala, maple syrup, and sea salt to the pan. Stir vigorously to combine, and turn the heat off after the liquid is absorbed by the pumpkin seeds.

- From here you can either let the pumpkin seeds cool in the pan, (if they stick to the pan use a metal spatula and they pop right out) or you can use them right away which adds a nice warm element to the salad.

- Toss the salad with the pumpkin seeds and vinaigrette.

- Serve immediately.

Cream Pancakes

TOTAL TIME: 25 MINUTES

INGREDIENTS

- 3 cups (426 g) all-purpose flour (see note for whole wheat flour)

- 2 tablespoons (27 g) granulated sugar

- 1 ½ teaspoons baking powder

- ¾ teaspoon baking soda

- ½ teaspoon salt

- 1 ½ cups (340 g) sour cream

- 1 ½ cups milk

- 3 large eggs (150 g out of shell)

- 6 tablespoons (85 g) butter, melted (see note)

Directions

- In a large bowl, whisk together the flour, sugar, baking powder, baking soda, and salt.

- In a separate bowl, whisk together the sour cream, milk, eggs and butter.

- Add the wet ingredients to the dry and mix with a spoon or spatula until just combined. The batter will be lumpy and it's ok if there are even a few streaks of flour here and there. Don't overmix! The key to light and fluffy pancakes is mixing just until combined.

- Let the batter rest while prepping the griddle.

- Heat a nonstick griddle to medium for 1-2 minutes until a drop of water sizzles (about 300 degrees F on my griddle, but every griddle will be a bit different).

- Pour batter into rounds on the preheated griddle.

- Cook until small bubbles appear on the surface and the edges are set, 1-3 minutes, depending on the heat of the griddle.

- Flip the pancakes and cook for another minute or so until golden and cooked through. Repeat with remaining batter.

- Serve immediately or keep warm in a 175 degree F oven for 15-20 minutes.

TOTAL TIME: 25 MINUTES

Ingredients

- 2 tablespoons cider vinegar
- 1 tablespoon canola oil
- 2 teaspoons finely chopped canned chipotle chile in adobo sauce
- ¼ teaspoon salt
- 2 cups shredded red cabbage
- 1 medium carrot, shredded
- ¼ cup chopped fresh cilantro
- 1 15-ounce can white beans, rinsed
- 1 ripe avocado
- ½ cup shredded sharp Cheddar cheese
- 2 tablespoons minced red onion
- 4 8- to 10-inch whole-wheat wraps, or tortillas

Directions

- Whisk vinegar, oil, chipotle chile and salt in a medium bowl. Add cabbage, carrot and cilantro; toss to combine.

- Mash beans and avocado in another medium bowl with a potato masher or fork. Stir in cheese and onion.

- To assemble the wraps, spread about 1/2 cup of the bean-avocado mixture onto a wrap (or tortilla) and top with about 2/3 cup of the cabbage-carrot slaw. Roll up. Repeat with remaining ingredients. Cut the wraps in half to serve, if desired.

Spinach and Eggs Scramble

TOTAL TIME: 20 MINUTES

Ingredients

- 2 tablespoons olive oil

- ½ medium onion sliced and separated into rings

- ½ teaspoon Diamond Crystal kosher salt plus a pinch for the onions

- ¼ teaspoon black pepper divided

- 4 large eggs

- 2 tablespoons grated Parmesan (1 oz)

- 2 cups fresh baby spinach leaves (2 oz)

- ¼ teaspoon red pepper flakes

Directions

- Heat a very large (12-14 inch) nonstick skillet over medium-high heat for about 2 minutes. Add the olive oil.

- Add the onion slices. Sprinkle them with a pinch of Kosher salt and a pinch of black pepper. Cook, stirring occasionally, until golden, about 5 minutes. Lower the heat to medium.

- While the onion is cooking, in a medium bowl, whisk together the eggs, ½ teaspoon of Kosher salt, a pinch of black pepper, and 2 tablespoons of Parmesan. Set aside.

- When the onions are golden brown, add the spinach leaves to the skillet. Cook, stirring, just until beginning to wilt, about 1 minute. Don't overcook the spinach at this point.

- Pour the egg mixture into the skillet. Cook the eggs over medium heat, pushing them back and forth with a rubber spatula, until set to your liking. Sprinkle with red pepper flakes. Serve immediately.

TOTAL TIME: 1 HOUR 15 MINUTES

Ingredients

- 400g / 14oz curly pasta , dried (or other of choice)
- 1/4 cup parsley , roughly chopped (or chives)
- 120g / 4oz feta , crumbled into big chunks
- 2 capsicum/bell peppers (1 red, 1 yellow), cut into 2.5cm / 1" pieces
- 1 red onion, cut into wedges
- 1 eggplant, halved lengthwise, then 1.25cm/ 0.5" thick semi circles
- 2 zucchini, cut into 1.5cm / 2/3" chunks (see video)
- 200g/ 7oz button mushrooms, halved (large ones quartered)
- 1 bunch asparagus, ends trimmed, cut into 5cm/2" lengths
- 1/4 cup (65ml) extra virgin olive oil
- 1 tsp each salt and pepper
- 3 cloves garlic, minced

- 1/3 cup (85ml) lemon juice

- 1/3 cup (85ml) extra virgin olive oil

- 2 tsp white sugar

- 2 garlic cloves, minced

- 1/2 tsp each salt and pepper

- 1/2 tsp each dried basil, parsley, oregano, thyme

- 1/2 – 1 tsp chilli flakes (adjust spice to taste)

Directions

- Place ingredients in a jar and shake well. Set aside 10 minutes.

- Preheat oven to 250°C/480°F (230°F fan).

- Place all vegetables other than asparagus in a large bowl. Drizzle with oil, sprinkle with salt, pepper and garlic, toss.

- Spread vegetables on 2 trays (fill one less than the other). Roast 25 minutes, tossing once.

- Drizzle asparagus with oil and pinch of salt and pepper. Add into oven for last 5 minutes.

- Transfer vegetables into large bowl, pour over 1/2 the Dressing. Toss, then leave to marinate for 30 minutes to 3 hours.

- In large pot of salted water, cook pasta per packet directions but add 2 minutes to the cook time (Note 5 for why). Drain and return pasta into pot.

- Add vegetables, including veg juices, into the pasta pot. Add remaining dressing and parsley, then toss. Set aside for 15 minutes to cool slightly.

- Serve! Sprinkle with feta and serve! Keeps 4 – 5 days, serve at room temp.

Quinoa Salad

TOTAL TIME: 25 MINUTES

Ingredients

- 3 1/2 cups leftover cooked quinoa (chilled)
- 1 large red bell pepper
- 2 cups diced English cucumber
- 1 1/2 cups grape tomatoes, halved

- 1 medium carrot, shredded (1/2 cup)

- 1/2 cup chopped red onion, rinsed under cold water in a sieve and drained

- 1 (14.5 oz) can chick peas, drained and rinsed

- 1/3 cup olive oil

- 3 Tbsp fresh lemon juice

- 2 Tbsp red wine vinegar

- 1/3 cup chopped fresh parsley (chop somewhat fine)

- 1/4 cup chopped fresh cilantro (chop somewhat fine)

- 2 garlic cloves, minced (2 tsp)

- Salt, to taste

Directions

- Roast red pepper directly over the flame of a gas stove or under broiler, turning occasionally using metal tongs, until charred all over. Transfer to a container and cover and let rest 10 minutes, then peel, core and seed and chop pepper.

- Meanwhile prepare dressing. In a mixing bowl stir together olive oil, lemon juice, red wine vinegar, parsley, cilantro, garlic and salt. Chill while you prep the remaining salad ingredients or up to 1 day.

- In large bowl toss together quinoa, pepper, cucumber, tomato, carrot, onion and chick peas with the dressing. Serve within about 4 hours for best results. Keep salad chilled.

Salmon with Lentil Salad

TOTAL TIME: 25 MINUTES

Ingredients

- 4 skinless salmon fillets, about 700 g total
- 3/4 tsp salt, divided
- 2 tbsp plus 2 tsp olive oil, divided
- 2 tbsp lemon juice
- 2 garlic cloves, minced
- 1 tsp sumac
- 1/2 tsp Dijon mustard
- 1 540-mL can lentils, drained and rinsed
- 1 pint multicoloured cherry tomatoes, halved
- 4 cups loosely packed stemmed arugula

- 1/2 cup chopped mint

- 1/2 cup chopped parsley

Directions

- Sprinkle salmon with 1⁄2 tsp salt. Season with pepper. Heat a large non-stick frying pan over medium-high. Add 2 tsp olive oil, and then salmon. Cook until underside of fillet is light-golden, 3 to 4 min. Turn fish over and continue cooking until a knife tip inserted in centre and held for 10 sec comes out warm, about 3 min more. Set aside.

- Whisk lemon juice with garlic, sumac, Dijon and remaining 2 tbsp oil and 1/4 tsp salt in a large bowl. Stir in lentils, cherry tomatoes, arugula, mint and parsley. Season with pepper. Toss to coat.

- Arrange lentil mixture on a platter. Top with salmon.

TOTAL TIME: 15 MINUTES

Ingredients

- 6 tablespoons mayonnaise (or plain yogurt)
- 1 tablespoon lemon juice
- 1/2 teaspoon kosher salt
- Pinch freshly ground black pepper
- 2 sweet apples, cored and chopped
- 1 cup seedless red grapes, halved, or 1/4 cup raisins
- 1 cup thinly sliced celery
- 1 cup chopped, slightly toasted walnuts
- Lettuce

Directions

- In a medium sized bowl, whisk together the mayonnaise (or yogurt), lemon juice, salt and pepper.
- Stir the apple, celery, grapes, and walnuts into the bowl with the dressing.

- Spoon salad onto a bed of fresh lettuce and serve.

Grilled Veggie & Steak Salad

TOTAL TIME: 30 MINUTES

Ingredients

- ½ cup red wine vinegar (120 mL)
- ½ teaspoon pepper
- ¼ teaspoon salt
- 1 teaspoon dried oregano
- 2 cloves garlic
- ¼ cup olive oil (59 mL)
- 1 zucchini
- 1 summer squash
- 1 small red onion
- 1 red bell pepper
- 1 yellow bell pepper
- 1 ½ lb ribeye steak (680 g)
- Salt, to taste
- Pepper, to taste

- 1 bag mixed greens salad

- Olive oil, to taste

- Red wine vinegar, to taste

- Salt, to taste

- Pepper, to taste

Directions

- Cut zucchini and summer squash in half lengthwise. Remove the insides of the bell peppers and cut into large chunks. Remove the top and bottom from the red onion and slice horizontally into three pieces.

- Combine red wine vinegar, pepper, salt, oregano, and garlic.

- Whisk in the olive oil and coat vegetables in the dressing. Place on a baking sheet.

- Season the rib eye with salt and pepper.

- Grill steak over medium-high heat for 5-7 minutes on each side (times may vary depending on the grill and how well-done you like your steak).

- Add the vegetables to the grill and cook the zucchini and summer squash for 5-7 minutes on each side. Cook the bell peppers and onions 4-6 minutes each side (times may vary depending on the grill).

- Remove steak from the grill and let rest for 10 minutes.

- Slice the steak into strips.

- Cut vegetables into small pieces. Arrange vegetables and steak on a bed of mixed greens.

- Drizzle olive oil, red wine vinegar, salt, and pepper over the salad. Enjoy!

Broccoli, Chard and Bean Soup

TOTAL TIME: 40 MINUTES

Ingredients

- 9 Chard Leaves coarsley chopped

- 3 Heads Broccoli cut into florets

- 4 Cloves Garlic minced

- 1 Yellow Onion chopped

- 1 15 Ounce Can Pinto Beans, drained and rinsed

- 2 and 3/4 cup chicken broth

- 2/3 Cup Grated Parmesan Cheese

- 2 Tablespoons Olive Oil

- 2 Teaspoons Fresh Rosemary chopped

- 1/2 Teaspoon Ground Black Pepper

- Salt if neccessary

Directions

- Steam the broccoli florets for 5 minutes. If you don't have steamer tray to put inside a pot, you can always use a small metal strainer, which is what I did. Set the broccoli aside.

- In a large pot, heat the garlic, onions, and rosemary in the olive oil until the onions are slightly transparent, stirring every minute or two for about 5 minutes. Add the beans and swiss chard and cover, cooking for another 5 minutes. Add the chicken broth and the pepper and bring the liquid to a boil, then cook the soup for about 7 minutes.

- Remove the soup from heat, add the broccoli and Parmesan cheese and stir. Ladle the soup into a food processor or blender and blend it until a smooth puree forms, about 1 minute. Depending upon the size of your blender or food processor, you may need to do blend the soup in batches, like I did. Taste and add some salt, if necessary.

- Serve hot with a sprinkle of Parmesan cheese and a decorative slice of chard stem.

Corn Chowder

TOTAL TIME: 1 HOUR 20 MINUTES

Ingredients

- 1 tablespoon butter
- 1 strip bacon, or 1 teaspoon bacon fat
- 1/2 large yellow onion, chopped (about 3/4 cup)
- 1/3 cup diced red bell pepper
- 1/2 cup small diced carrot
- 1/2 cup small diced celery
- 4 to 5 ears sweet corn, kernels removed from the cobs (about 3 cups), cobs reserved
- 1 bay leaf

- 4 1/2 cups milk, whole or low fat

- 2 medium Yukon Gold potatoes, peeled and large (1-inch) diced (about 3 cups)

- 1 tablespoon kosher salt

- 1/2 teaspoon freshly ground black pepper

- 1 teaspoon fresh thyme leaves

Directions

- Place butter and bacon into a large, heavy-bottomed soup pot. Heat on medium heat until the bacon renders its fat, 3-4 minutes.

- Add the chopped onions, red bell pepper, carrot, and celery, lower the heat to medium low and cook until vegetables soften, about 5 minutes.

- Break the corn cobs in half (after you've stripped off the corn) and add the cobs to the pot. Add the milk and the bay leaf. Bring to a boil and reduce heat to a bare simmer. Cover the pot and cook for 20 minutes.

- Make sure the heat is as low as can be and still maintain a gentle simmer (on our stove we had to use the "warm" setting) to prevent scalding the milk on the bottom of the pan.

- After 20 minutes, add the potatoes, salt, and thyme to the pot. Increase the heat to return the soup to a simmer, then lower the heat to maintain the simmer and cook for another 10 minutes.

- Discard the cobs, the bacon strip, and the bay leaf. Add the corn kernels and black pepper. Again raise the heat to bring the soup to a simmer, then lower the heat and cook for another 5 minutes, until the potatoes are fork tender.

Chickpea Harissa Vegetable Soup

TOTAL TIME: 40 MINUTES

Ingredients

- 1 tablespoon olive oil
- 1 small yellow onion roughly chopped
- 2 carrots peeled and diced
- 1 red bell pepper diced

- 2 garlic cloves minced

- 3 tablespoons harissa

- 1 teaspoon cumin

- 1/2 teaspoon paprika

- 1 teaspoon kosher salt

- 1/2 teaspoon black pepper

- 1-28 ounce can crushed tomatoes

- 4 cups low-sodium vegetable broth

- 1 cup water

- 2 medium zucchini diced

- 1-14.5 ounce can chickpeas drained and rinsed

- Chopped fresh parsley for serving

Directions

- Heat the oil in a large saucepan over medium heat. Add the onions and carrots and sauté for 4 minutes until the onions start to soften. Add the peppers and continue cooking for 2-3 minutes.

- Add the garlic, harissa, cumin, paprika, salt and pepper and sauté for 1-2 minutes until fragrant.

- Pour in the tomatoes, vegetable broth and water and bring the mixture to a boil. Reduce the heat and simmer for 10 minutes.

- Add the zucchini and chickpeas and continue simmering for 10 minutes, letting the soup thicken slightly.

- Divide the soup into bowls and top with chopped parsley before serving.

Mushroom and Thyme Cream Soup

TOTAL TIME: 30 MINUTES

Ingredients

- 1 Tablespoon extra virgin olive oil

- ¾ pound (335 g) wild mushrooms, sliced

- 2 Tablespoons fresh thyme leaves

- 1 (75 g) medium shallot, peeled, sliced

- 1 cup (155 g) raw cashews

- 4 cups (960 ml) vegetable stock

- ½ teaspoon sea salt

Directions

- In a large skillet over medium-high heat, add the olive oil, mushrooms, fresh thyme leaves, and shallot and sauté until softened, about 10 minutes.

- Place vegetable stock, cashews, and sautéed mixture into the Vitamix container in the order listed and secure the lid.

- Start the blender on its lowest speed, then quickly increase to its highest speed. Blend for 5 minutes 45 seconds; or select the Hot Soup program and allow the machine to complete the programmed cycle

Stuffed Acorn Squash

TOTAL TIME: 1 HOUR

Ingredients

- 2 acorn squash, halved

- 1 (8-ounce) package tempeh

- 1 tablespoon extra-virgin olive oil, more for drizzling

- ½ yellow onion, chopped

- 8 ounces cremini mushrooms, diced

- 3 garlic cloves, minced

- ⅓ cup coarsely chopped walnuts

- 1 tablespoon tamari

- 1 tablespoon apple cider vinegar

- ½ tablespoon chopped rosemary

- ¼ cup chopped sage

- ⅓ cup dried cranberries

- Parsley and a few pomegranate arils, for garnish

- Sea salt and freshly ground black pepper

Directions

- Preheat the oven to 425°F and line a baking sheet with parchment paper. Scoop out and discard the seeds from the squash. Place the squash halves on the baking sheet, and drizzle them with olive oil and pinches of salt and pepper. Roast cut-side up for 40 minutes, or until tender.

- While the squash roasts, cut the tempeh into ½-inch cubes, place in a steamer basket, and set over a pot filled with 1 inch of water. Bring the water to a simmer, cover the pot, and steam for 10 minutes. Remove, drain any excess water, and use your hands to crumble the tempeh.

- Heat the olive oil in a large skillet over medium heat. Add the onion, ½ teaspoon salt, and several grinds of black pepper and cook 5 minutes. Add the mushrooms and cook, stirring, until soft, about 8 minutes.

- Stir in the crumbled tempeh, garlic, walnuts, tamari, apple cider vinegar, rosemary, and sage and cook 2 to 3 minutes more, adding ¼ cup water as the pan gets dry.

- Stir in the cranberries and season to taste. Scoop the filling into the roasted acorn squash halves and garnish with the parsley and pomegranates.

Tofu Quinoa

Ingredients

- 1 block extra firm tofu
- 1 tablespoon extra virgin olive oil
- 2 tablespoon soy sauce, low-sodium
- 1 tablespoon cornstarch
- ½ teaspoon garlic powder
- ¼ teaspoon ground ginger
- 1 large sweet potato
- 1 small red onion
- 3 cups kale, packed
- 1 tablespoon extra virgin olive oil
- ¼ teaspoon salt
- ¼ teaspoon pepper
- 1 cup quinoa, uncooked
- 2 cups vegetable broth, low-sodium
- 1 avocado
- 3 teaspoon chia seeds

Directions

- Drain the tofu block. Slice it into two flat slabs. Press them for 15 minutes by lining them with a kitchen towel and placing something heavy on them such as a pan.

- Preheat the oven to 400°F and line a large sheet pan with a nonstick mat or parchment paper.

- Slice the tofu slabs into cubes and add them to a bowl that has a fitted lid or a gallon bag. Add a tablespoon of olive oil and soy sauce. Close the bowl and shake it till the cubes are fully coated. Let this marinade absorb while preparing the other veggies.

- Peel and cut the sweet potato into 1-inch cubes. Cut the red onion into chunks. Add them to the sheet pan along with the kale. Leave a fourth of the sheet pan empty for the tofu.

- Mix the garlic powder and ginger with the cornstarch, then sprinkle it over the tofu. Close the bowl back up and shake it around gently until the cubes are fully coated. Place the tofu cubes on the sheet pan in a single layer.

- Drizzle the vegetables with olive oil, and then sprinkle salt and pepper over everything, including the tofu.

- Roast the tofu and veggies for 30 minutes in the oven. Flip everything halfway through. Add more olive oil if anything looks like it's drying out and remove any veggies that look like they might burn.

- Cook the quinoa while the other ingredients are roasting. You may need to rinse your quinoa if the package doesn't say "pre-rinsed." Bring the quinoa and broth to a boil in a medium pot. Then, reduce the heat to a simmer. Cover the pot and cook the quinoa for 15 minutes. Fluff the quinoa with a fork once all of the broth is absorbed.

- Make the optional spicy tahini sauce by whisking the sauce ingredients together. (The recipe is down below in the notes section.)

- Divide everything across five bowls with the quinoa as the base. Top them with avocado slices, chia seeds, and sauce. Enjoy these tofu power bowls now or save them for later!

Spicy Honey Chicken

TOTAL TIME: 25 MINUTES

Ingredients

- 8 boneless skinless chicken thighs, about 2 pounds
- 2 teaspoons vegetable oil
- 2 teaspoons granulated garlic
- 2 teaspoons chili powder
- 1/2 teaspoon onion powder
- 1/2 teaspoon coriander
- 1 teaspoon kosher salt
- 1 teaspoon cumin
- 1/2 teaspoon chipotle chili powder
- 1/2 cup honey
- 1 tablespoon cider vinegar

Directions

- Combine the rub spices in bowl and mix well.

- Use kitchen shears (or a pair of clean scissors) to trim off any excess fat from the chicken pieces. Pat dry. Drizzle oil over chicken and rub in with your hands to lightly coat all the pieces. Then toss chicken with the spice rub to coat all sides well. Use your hands and get in there! Grill chicken for 3-5 minutes on each side, until cooked through.

- While chicken is cooking, warm honey in the microwave so it's not so thick. Add the vinegar and combine well. Reserve 2 tablespoons honey glaze for later. Take the rest and brush on chicken (both sides) in the final moments of grilling.

TOTAL TIME: 60 MINUTES

Ingredients

- 3 tablespoons butter
- 1 leek, thinly sliced (white and green parts only)
- 2 cups diced carrots
- 1 cup diced celery
- 3-4 cloves garlic, minced
- 3 tablespoons flour
- 6 cups chicken or vegetable broth
- 1 teaspoon oregano
- 1 teaspoon thyme
- 2 cups cubed butternut squash
- 1 cup wild rice
- 3 cups spinach, chopped
- 2-3 cups cooked, cubed turkey
- 2 cups heavy cream
- 2 tablespoons chopped fresh parsley
- Salt and pepper, to taste

Directions

- In a large Dutch oven, melt butter over medium heat. Add the leeks, carrots, celery and garlic and cook until vegetables are soft, about 5-8 minutes.

- Add the flour and continue to cook and stir for another 1-2 minutes. Slowly whisk in the broth and bring to a simmer.

- Stir in the oregano, thyme, squash and wild rice. Continue cooking for another 20-25 minutes, until the squash is tender and the rice is cooked.

- Stir in the spinach and cooked turkey, along with the cream and parsley. Bring to a simmer and season with salt and pepper, to taste.

Coconut Lemongrass Scallops with Lime

TOTAL TIME: 25 MINUTES

Ingredients

- 1 shallot, finely diced
- 4 tablespoons white vinegar
- 1 stalk of fresh lemongrass (about 4–5 inches), smashed
- 2 thin slices ginger (optional)
- 14-ounce can coconut milk (full fat is best here)
- 1 large lime – zest and juice
- 1 1/2 teaspoons fish sauce, plus more to taste
- few slices red chili (optional)
- 1 – 1 ¼ pound large scallops (about 4 ounces per person, or 3–4 large scallops)
- 1 tablespoon coconut oil for searing (or vegetable oil)
- salt and pepper
- 8 leaves of fresh basil (cut into thin ribbons)

Directions

- Put a small pot of rice to cook on stove. In a small sauce pan, simmer shallot in vinegar on low heat, until vinegar reduces almost completely, about 5 minutes.

- Add coconut milk, ½ of the lime zest (save the rest for garnish) the smashed lemongrass and the ginger, and simmer gently on medium low heat for 5 minutes. Do not over boil. Stir in 1 ½ teaspoons fish sauce and 1 tablespoon lime juice, turn the heat off and taste. Adjust with more lime or fish sauce if you want. Add a few slices of fresh red chili for heat. Set aside and let flavors infuse while the rice is cooking.

- Gently rinse and pat dry scallops. Season with salt and pepper.

- In a skillet, heat coconut oil over medium heat. When the skillet is hot add the scallops and sear each side 2-3 minutes (depending on the size). When done to your liking, set aside and give a little squeeze of lime. When ready to serve, warm up the sauce just a bit, and strain.

- Assemble the bowls. Divide rice, top with scallops, then spoon the flavorful lemongrass coconut sauce over top, garnishing with fresh basil ribbons and remaining lime zest. Enjoy!

Cashew Crusted Fish Tacos

TOTAL TIME: 30 MINUTES

Ingredients

- 1 lb cod sliced into half-inch thick strips, 1 to 2 inches in length
- 8 oz lightly salted roasted whole cashews
- ¼ cup fresh parsley finely chopped
- ½ tsp ground sage
- 1 tsp salt
- 1 tsp black pepper
- 2 large eggs
- 1 to 2 tbsp water

- ½ cup mayo

- ½ to 1 lemon juiced

- 2 tsp fresh parsley finely chopped

- ½ tsp roasted garlic powder

- ⅛ tsp ground sage

- ⅛ tsp dill weed

- ¼ tsp salt

- ¼ head red cabbage thinly sliced

- ½ lemon juiced

- 2 pinches sea salt

- 12 corn tortillas 4-inch

- Finely chopped fresh parsley optional garnish

- 4 lemon wedges optional garnish

Directions

- Preheat oven to 425 degrees. Line a large baking sheet with parchment paper and lightly grease with cooking spray.

- Prepare the cashew crust. Add cashews to a food processor and crush into a breadcrumb-like powder, then transfer to a shallow dish.

Add chopped parsley, ground sage, salt and pepper and stir to combine. Set aside.

- Prepare the egg wash. Whisk together eggs and water in a shallow dish until combined, then set aside.

- Coat the sliced cod in the egg wash, then transfer to the cashew crust and coat well. Lay fish strips flat on the baking sheet, spacing them at least a half-inch apart.

- Lightly grease the fish with cooking spray, then bake for 10 minutes or until cashew crust is lightly browned and fish is cooked through.

- Next, prepare the lemon herb aioli. Add all ingredients to a small bowl and whisk until well-combined and the consistency is creamy and pourable, but not too thin. Refrigerate until ready to serve.

- Finally, prepare the quick pickled cabbage. Add thinly sliced red cabbage to a large bowl and season with lemon juice and sea salt. Gently toss to combine and let rest for about 10 minutes before serving.

- Once all the components are ready, assemble the tacos. Warm the tortillas on a skillet over medium-high heat or in the microwave, then fill each with a few strips of fish, a drizzle of lemon herb aioli, and a handful of cabbage. Optionally garnish with fresh chopped parsley and a lemon wedge. Serve immediately.

Pumpkin Pudding

TOTAL TIME: 60 MINUTES

Ingredients

- 3/4 cup granulated sugar
- 1 teaspoon ground cinnamon
- 1/2 teaspoon ground ginger
- 1/2 teaspoon kosher salt
- 1/4 teaspoon ground cloves
- 2 large eggs
- 1 (15-ounce) can pumpkin purée
- 1 (12-ounce) can evaporated milk
- Whipped cream, for serving (optional)

Directions

- Heat the oven to 350°F. In a small bowl, mix the sugar, cinnamon, ginger, salt, and cloves.

- In a large bowl, beat the eggs to blend. Stir in the pumpkin purée and sugar-spice mixture. Gradually stir in the evaporated milk.

- Pour into glass or ceramic baking dish. A good thing to know is that you can fill a baking dish deeper than a pie crust, but it's best not to exceed a depth of about 1½ inches. Baking times vary with the depth, size, and type of baking dish, so you just have to watch and check. Bake until a knife inserted near the center comes out clean. Let cool on wire rack, then refrigerate overnight, until ready to serve. Serve with the whipped cream, if using.

TOTAL TIME: 15 MINUTES

Ingredients

- 2 cups whole milk
- ½ cup sugar
- ¼ cup cocoa powder
- 4 teaspoons cornstarch
- 2 large egg yolks
- 2 teaspoons pure vanilla extract
- ¼ teaspoon salt
- ½ cup dark chocolate chopped
- 2 tablespoons butter

Directions

- In a saucepan, whisk together the milk, sugar, cocoa powder, cornstarch, egg yolks, vanilla, and salt. Cook over medium-high heat whisking constantly, until the mixture comes to a simmer. Add the chocolate and butter.

- While continuing to constantly mix, bring to a full boil. Reduce the heat to maintain a simmer, and continue whisking until thick, about 2 or 3 minutes more.

- Pour the pudding into 6 small cups or ramekins. Place a piece of plastic wrap directly onto the pudding and refrigerate for at least 4 hours or until set.

Grilled Beef Tenderloin Filets with Chimichurri Sauce

TOTAL TIME: 30 MINUTES

Ingredients

- 1½ tablespoons paprika
- 1½ teaspoons ground cumin
- 1½ teaspoons ground mustard (also called dry mustard)
- 1 teaspoon coarsely ground black pepper
- 1½ teaspoons kosher salt
- 6 tablespoons extra virgin olive oil

- 1½ tablespoons Sherry wine vinegar (or red wine vinegar)

- 1½ tablespoons fresh lemon juice, from 1 lemon

- 2 small garlic cloves, peeled and roughly chopped

- 1 medium shallot, peeled and roughly chopped

- ½ teaspoon salt

- ¼ teaspoon freshly ground black pepper

- ¼ teaspoon crushed red pepper flakes

- 1½ cups stemmed fresh parsley

- 1 cup stemmed fresh cilantro

- ½ cup stemmed fresh mint

- 4 (6-8 ounce) beef tenderloin filets (about 1-inch thick)

- 2 tablespoons olive oil

Directions

- Combine all of the ingredients in a small bowl and stir until well combined.

- Combine the olive oil, wine vinegar, lemon juice, garlic cloves, shallot, salt, pepper, red pepper flakes and a third of the herbs in a blender; blend until almost smooth. Add the remaining herbs in two separate additions, puréeing until almost smooth after each addition. Cover and chill until ready to serve.

- Remove the tenderloin filets from the refrigerator and let sit at room temperature for about 30 minutes. Preheat the grill to high (about 600 degrees).

- Drizzle the filets with the olive oil and rub until evenly coated. Sprinkle the spice rub all over the filets and pat down with your hands so it sticks (the coating will be thick).

- Clean and oil the cooking grate. Place the filets on the grill and cook, covered, about 4 minutes, or until nicely browned and charred on the first side. Flip the steaks and cook 3-4 minutes more for medium-rare. Transfer to a platter, tent with foil and let rest for 5-10 minutes. Serve the filets with chimichurri sauce on the side.